CHINESE HEALTH QIGONG

Taiji Yangsheng Zhang

Taiji Stick Qigong

T0271807

CHINESE HEALTH QIGONG ASSOCIATION

The accompanying online materials can be downloaded at
https://library.singingdragon.com/redeem using the code VOUFYKY

This edition published in 2014
by Singing Dragon
an imprint of Jessica Kingsley Publishers
73 Collier Street
London N1 9BE, UK
and
400 Market Street, Suite 400
Philadelphia, PA 19106, USA

www.singingdragon.com

First published by Foreign Languages Press, Beijing, China, 2012

Copyright © Foreign Languages Press 2012, 2014

Library of Congress Cataloging in Publication Data
A CIP catalog record for this book is available from the Library of Congress

British Library Cataloguing in Publication Data
A CIP catalogue record for this book is available from the British Library

ISBN 978 1 78775 235 1

Printed and bound by CPI Group (UK) Ltd, Croydon, CR0 4YY

CONTENTS

The accompanying online materials can be downloaded at
https://library.singingdragon.com/redeem using the code VOUFYKY

CHAPTER 1

Origins

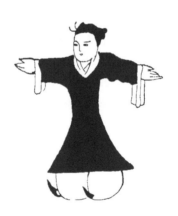

Sticks are among the tools first used by human beings. In China's traditional health culture, it has long been a practice to exercise with an instrument like a stick. In the *Pictures of Daoyin Exercises* excavated from the Mawangdui Tomb of the Han Dynasty (206 BC–AD 220) in Changsha of Hunan Province, there are two illustrations of figures in different postures wielding sticks (Figs. 1 and 2). They are by far the earliest document to teach people how to keep fit by stick exercises.

From the earliest time "dance" meant to ward off disease and keep fit, to various other health preservation methods such as *daoyin* (Chinese traditional fitness exercise which combines breath control, body and limb movements, concentration of mind, and local massage), we see a form of exercise with the stick as an instrument.

According to historical records, the *Book of Zhuangzi* wrote, "exhaling and inhaling, or imitating a bear climbing a tree and a bird reaching out its feet – they are all about regimens..." Regimens have combined *daoyin* with *qi*-regulating exercises.

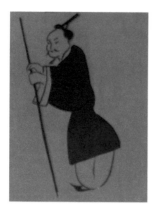

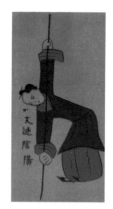

Fig. 1   Fig. 2

The *Huang Di Nei Jing* (Yellow Emperor's Medicine) explains, "The land in the center is flat and wet, and all things grew there. Its people ate everything and did not much labor. So most people were affected by numbness of limbs, faintness, cold and heat, and their best treatment was *daoyin* (导引) and massage." A large number of historical records and the use of the stick mentioned in the *Pictures of Daoyin Exercises* indicate a relationship between body building, breathing exercises and other fitness methods in ancient China. This is the intellectual basis for us to identify, adapt and create new body-building regimens. The *Pictures of Daoyin Exercises* and the modern Taiji Stick (*Taiji Yangsheng Zhang*) show that the regimen using the stick has a long history, and this practice continues till today.

Based on the *Pictures of Daoyin Exercises,* this book creates a new Taiji Stick regimen based on the principles of *daoyin,* conscious breathing and the successful experience of traditional practice methods with instruments such as the Taiji Stick.

CHAPTER II

Characteristics

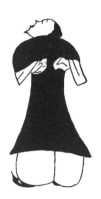

The Taiji Stick Health Preservation Exercises embodies the concept of harmony between *yin* and *yang*, man and nature. All the movements involved are soft and slow, and easy to practice. This is not a "martial art," *per se*, and the stick is not wielded like a weapon. The key points for the general practice of the Taiji Stick are as follows:

1. The Stick Guides Coordination of Body and Spirit

As the vehicle of human life, our body is a dynamic whole of flesh and blood, muscles, nerves and bones, meridian channels, and internal organs. In contrast, spirit, which dominates human life, refers to mental activities such as thought and concentration of the mind.

External matters include posture, body movements and ways to hold and use the stick; our internal focus encompasses breathing, thought, strength and vision.

The concept of our Taiji Stick regimen is to guide our breathing with the stick, giving first priority to attaining mental tranquility, and building up our bodies at the same time. Breathing should synchronize with our body movements, guided by the stick. When wielding the stick, we should ease our minds, let thoughts govern breathing, and harmonize body and spirit.

2. The Waist Functions as a Pivot to Harmonize the Body and the Stick

In practicing with the Taiji Stick, we should twist, turn, bend, and stretch around the waist as a center, and move our spine accordingly.

In practicing with the Taiji Stick, we need to relax our waist and hips, and keep the body upright and comfortable, adjusting the movement of the waist in harmony with use of the stick. If we lift the stick, we need to sink the waist and lower the *qi* down to the *Dantian* (lower belly); and, if we lower the stick, we need to straighten the waist and pull up the *qi* to the *Baihui* acupoint. If we rotate the stick in a circle, our waist becomes the anchor, moving our body and arms. All this illustrates the pivotal role of the waist.

3. Relationship of Stick Movement and Massage

The stick should not only guide coordination of your body movements and breathing, but should also help stretch muscles and strengthen bones, massage acupoints, clear meridian channels and activate internal organs. If we move the stick and massage our abdomen in exercise, we can further stimulate the internal organs, thus strengthening the stick's body-building effects.

4. Rotating the Stick

The path of the stick should be a coherent rotation, either horizontally, vertically or in any arc in between.

5. Hands and Stick are Integrated into One

As an extension of the arms, the stick becomes a part of the exerciser. In practice, hold the stick and guide the body movements with your waist as the center, and at the same time use the stick's motion to pull and push your internal organs, in harmony with each other.

This set of exercises is both suitable for use as a whole regimen and on an individual or selective basis. With our body motion guided by the stick, and particularly through rotating our wrists and spinal column and stretching the upper back and shoulders, we can stimulate the circulation of *qi* and blood and relax muscles and bones to balance *yin* and *yang*, keeping fit and healthy.

CHAPTER III

Key Points

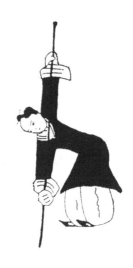

Section I Introduction to the Stick

The stick can be made of materials such as the branches of the white wax tree (*fraxinus*), pine tree and bamboo, which are smooth and even, or carved into auspicious patterns or with text about health. The size of the stick should be determined according to the height of the exerciser and by the size of his/her hands. The stick is usually 105 to 125 cm long and 2.3 to 2.8 cm in diameter (Figs. 3 to 5). (Both ends of the stick are carved with auspicious cloud images, but the patterns on the middle of the stick could differ.)

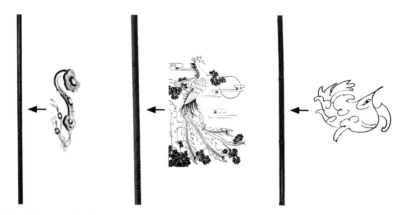

Fig. 3 Pine wood stick carved with *ruyi* pattern

Fig. 4 Pine wood stick carved with phoenix pattern

Fig. 5 Bamboo stick carved with *tianbao* pattern

Section II Basic Hand Positions and Wielding Methods

1. Basic Hand Positions

1) Holding the stick

Apply forefinger pressure to the stick, with the other fingers holding naturally around it (Fig. 6).

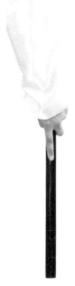

Fig. 6

2) *Grasping the stick*

Grasp the stick with cupped hands, pressing the thumbs lightly against the first joints of the forefingers (Fig. 7).

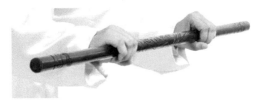

Fig. 7

3) *Clamping the stick*

Hold the stick against the *Hegu* acupoint between thumb and index finger and relax the hands, fingertips extended slightly upward, or, alternatively, flat, supporting the stick with your thumbs. See Fig. 10 for the vertical grip (Figs. 8 to 10).

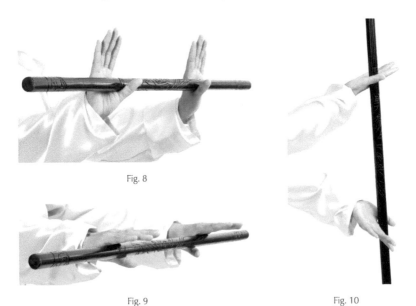

Fig. 8

Fig. 9   Fig. 10

4) Supporting the stick from beneath

Hold the stick on your open palms (Fig. 11).

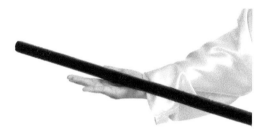

Fig. 11

2. Basic Wielding Methods

1) Rolling the stick

Grasp the stick and rotate the wrists forward (Fig. 12).

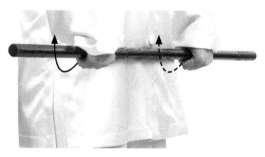

Fig. 12

2) Spinning the stick

Hold the stick pointed down at 45 degrees, with cupped hands, and rotate till one palm turns up. The other hand should adjust to this movement (Figs. 13 and 14).

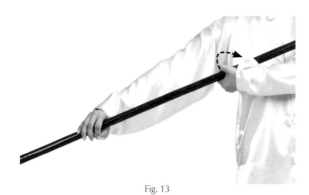

Fig. 13

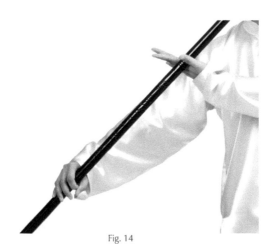

Fig. 14

3) Rotating the stick

Press the stick into *Hukou* acupoints between thumb and index finger with palms up. The hand close to one end of the stick rotates the wrist clockwise, and the second hand supports and cups the stick, with the stick rotating 90 degrees and rising to vertical (Figs. 15 to 17).

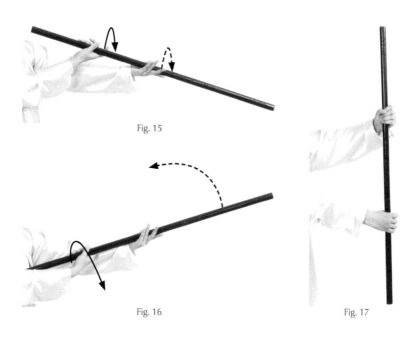

Fig. 15

Fig. 16

Fig. 17

4) Sliding the stick

One hand grips the horizontal stick and the other hand slides outward along it as the stick is raised (with the right hand as shown, Figs. 18 to 21).

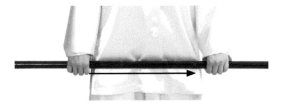

Fig. 18

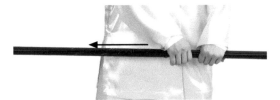

Fig. 19

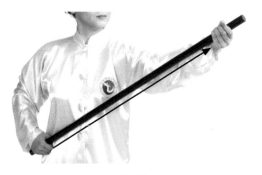

Fig. 20

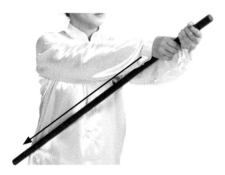

Fig. 21

5) Twisting the stick

One hand holds one end of the stick, drawing a circle high, then low and in toward your body, and finishing with one palm up, one down (with the right hand as shown, Figs. 22 and 23).

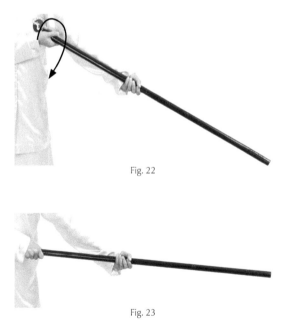

Fig. 22

Fig. 23

6) *Massage*

Hold the stick with arms shoulder-width apart, and then massage the body with the stick (abdominal and leg massage shown as example, Figs. 24 to 26).

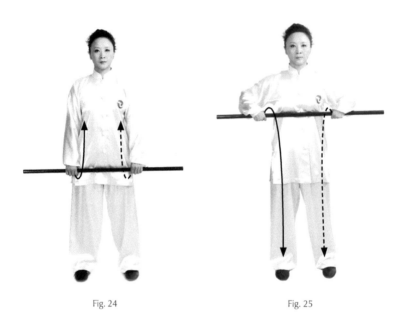

Fig. 24   Fig. 25

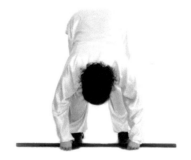

Fig. 26

Section III Basic Stances

1. Forward Stance

Step one leg out and bend it, with the lower leg vertical and toes facing front, but turning slightly inward. The other leg extends naturally with the foot standing firm, weight on the heel of the foot. The distance between feet is shoulder-width (Fig. 27).

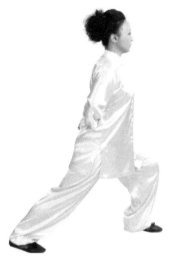

Fig. 27

2. High Squat

Cross your legs from behind, bend your knees and squat to press the *Chengshan* acupoint of the front leg with the rear leg (Fig. 28).

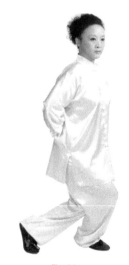

Fig. 28

3. Low Squat

Cross your legs from behind, then bend knees and squat until the hips rest on the heels. Hands are held behind the lower back. (Fig. 29).

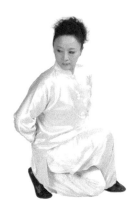

Fig. 29

Section IV Breathing and Concentrating the Mind

1. Breathing

Beginners should breathe naturally as needed, and as skills and mastery of each move advance, they can gradually learn abdominal breathing. The coordination of movements and breathing follows some basic principles – when moving upward, we move the stick away from the body and inhale; and when moving downward, we move the stick close to the body and exhale. Or when rolling the stick inward we inhale, and when rolling the stick outward we exhale.

2. Concentrating the Mind

The Taiji Stick regimen is characterized by the integration of meanings and forms, which change as your movement changes. In this process, you will become totally engrossed in yourself. In this way, the exerciser will relax and focus on the essentials of the exercise, concentrating the mind, form and breathing into one.

Section V Basic Training

1. Rolling the Stick

Stand naturally, grasp the stick and hold it in front of your abdomen. Your hands are shoulder-width apart; now rotate your wrists inward and outward (Figs. 30 and 31).

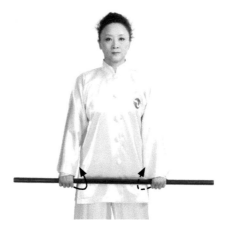

Fig. 30

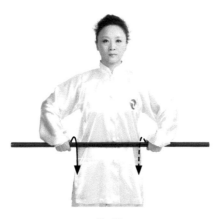

Fig. 31

2. Rotating the Stick

Stand naturally, grasp the stick and hold it in front of your abdomen. Your hands are shoulder-width apart. One arm rotates outward, until the palm is turned up, and then rotates back. The other hand coordinates its move. Alternate your active arm in practice (Figs. 32 and 33).

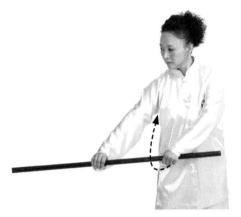

Fig. 32

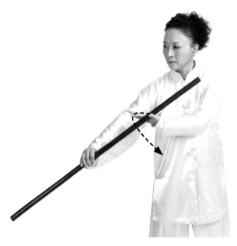

Fig. 33

3. Sliding the Stick

Stand upright, hold the stick in front of your abdomen with right palm up and left down. Your hands should be shoulder-width apart. Turn the stick upright with the right hand moving up and left hand moving down (Figs. 34 and 35). At the same time, both hands slide toward each other along the stick, and hold the stick, rotating the stick 180 degrees, with left palm facing up and right palm down, and bring the stick back in front of the abdomen (Figs. 36 and 37). Practice it in opposite direction.

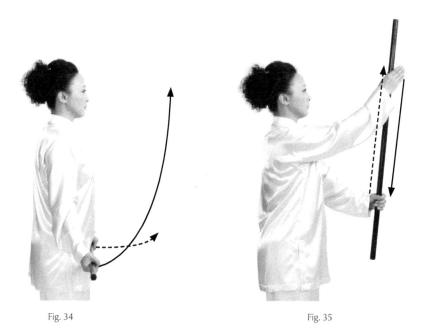

Fig. 34   Fig. 35

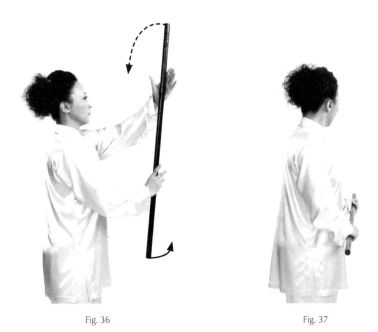

Fig. 36   Fig. 37

4. Drawing Circles

1) Horizontal circle

Use "drawing a circle to the left side" as an example. Bend your knees slightly with your feet shoulder-width apart. Turn to the left at the waist and at the same time clench the stick into the *Hegu* acupoints between thumb and index finger. Relax the fingers and, palm down, draw a wide circle from right to left (Figs. 38 to 40). Then stand upright, hold the stick and draw it in close to your abdomen to finish (Fig. 41). You can draw circles repeatedly in the same direction or the other direction.

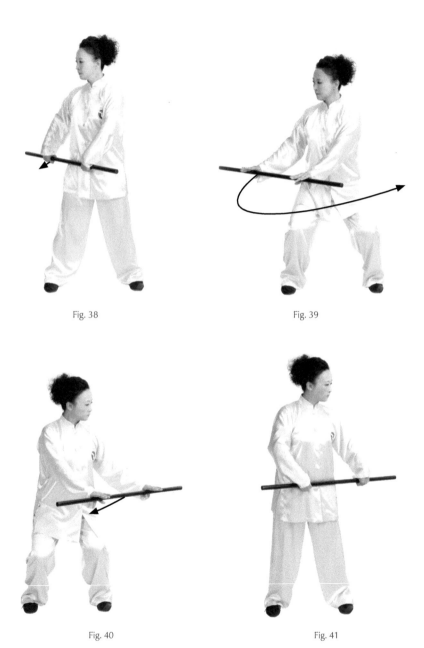

Fig. 38

Fig. 39

Fig. 40

Fig. 41

2) Vertical circle

Step one foot forward, bend your knees; with both hands holding the stick, wield it from the side to the rear, overhead and frontward until a full circle is completed. Then repeat this motion in the other direction (Figs. 42 to 45).

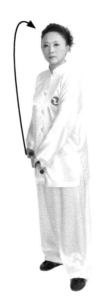

Fig. 42

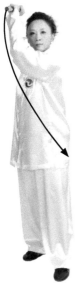

Fig. 43

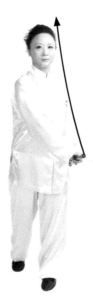

Fig. 44

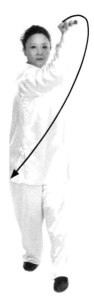

Fig. 45

Use "drawing a circle to your left side" as an example. The feet are shoulder-width apart. Hold the stick in front of your abdomen, and draw a circle from the right side, then upward, and overhead, downward to the left side (Figs. 46 to 48). Practice repeatedly in the same direction or the opposite direction.

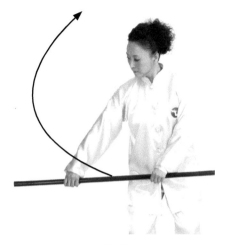

Fig. 46

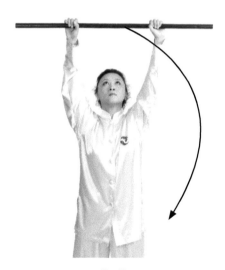

Fig. 47

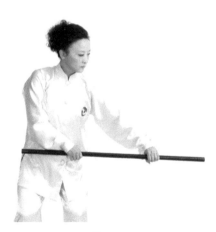

Fig. 48

5. Massage the Acupuncture Points

1) *Dazhui acupoint*

Stand upright, hold the stick in both hands and put it on your shoulders, then roll it with open palms up your neck from the *Dazhui* to the *Yuzhen* acupoints and back again (Figs. 49 and 50).

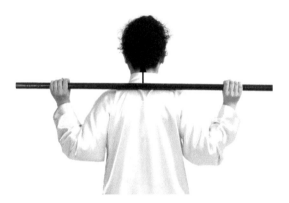

Fig. 49

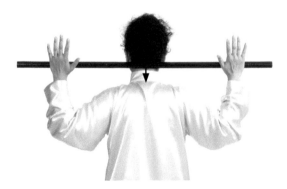

Fig. 50

2) *Jianjing acupoint*

Stand upright, hold the stick in both hands and put it on your shoulders. You may turn your waist to either side and at the same time press the *Jianjing* acupoints on the shoulders.

3) *Chengshan acupoint*

Cross your legs from behind, squat and press the *Chengshan* acupoint of the front leg with back leg (Figs. 51 and 52). If the right leg is forward, the left arm is raised and holding the stick high. Repeat the practice with the alternate leg and arm.

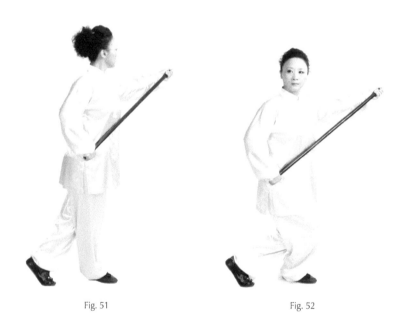

Fig. 51   Fig. 52

Movements

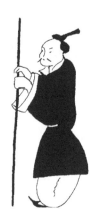

Section I Names of the Movements

Initial Stance
Step 1 Boatman Rows with an Oar (*Shao Gong Yao Lu*)
Step 2 Boat Rows Slowly (*Qing Zhou Huan Xing*)
Step 3 Wind Kisses Lotus Leaves (*Feng Bai He Ye*)
Step 4 Boatman Tows a Boat (*Chuan Fu Bei Qian*)
Step 5 Iron Stick Calms the Sea (*Shen Zhen Ding Hai*)
Step 6 Golden Dragon Wags Its Tail (*Jin Long Jiao Wei*)
Step 7 Search for Treasure in the Sea (*Tan Hai Xun Bao*)
Step 8 *Qi* Returns to *Dantian* (*Qi Gui Dan Tian*)
Ending Stance

Section II Movements, Tips and Health Benefits

Initial Stance

Movements

1. Stand upright, and keep your feet together with the whole body relaxed; hold the stick with the left hand about one third of its length from one end, with the stick extending up and behind your left arm. Let your arms hang naturally at your sides. Look straight ahead and be calm (Fig. 53).

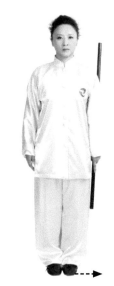

Fig. 53

2. Step your left foot to the side to shoulder-width from the right and stand erect. Raise the lower tip of the stick with your left hand and taking it in your right hand, slide it across the abdomen. Hold the stick with hands shoulder-width apart and look straight ahead (Fig. 54).

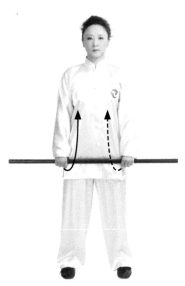

Fig. 54

3. Roll the stick up over the abdomen to the chest, and then back down till your arms are straight, and look straight ahead (Figs. 55 and 56).

Repeat twice.

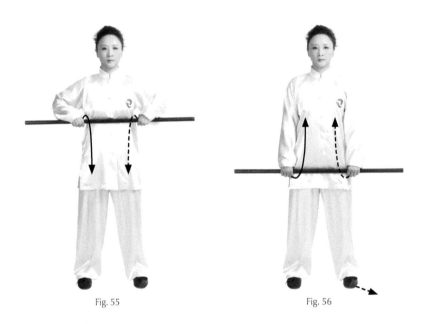

Fig. 55   Fig. 56

Tips

1. When you stand, keep your legs straight and body upright. Consciously lift your *Baihui* acupoint, draw back your chin slightly, lower your shoulders, relax your waist, pull up your hips, hold your breath, and concentrate your mind.

2. When you roll the stick upward, you should turn your wrists and elbows and move the stick all at the same time, inhaling accordingly. Then roll the stick downward, move your wrists and arms, and exhale accordingly.

Health benefits

1. Guiding the movements with your stick will calm your mind, relax your body, and keep your mind concentrated.

2. Coordination of breathing and movements helps you to get rid of stale *qi* and take in fresh air.

Step 1 Boatman Rows with an Oar (*Shao Gong Yao Lu*)
Movements

1. Continue from the Initial stance. Bend your knees, hold the stick chest-high, and with your left foot step 45 degrees to the front and left. Arch your toes up and keep your heel close to the ground as you step out. Turn your body 45 degrees to the left, and roll the stick back to your chest, turning your wrists and elbows (Fig. 57). Then settle your left foot, shift your weight forward into a left bow stance, and at the same time, clamp the stick and push it upward,

forward and then downward until it ends at waist height, as if you were rowing with an oar. Eyes follow the direction of the stick (Figs. 58 and 59).

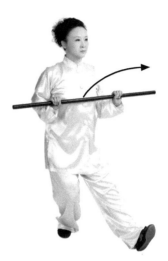

Fig. 57

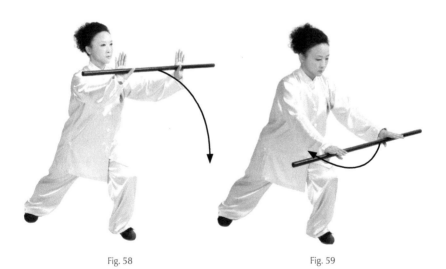

Fig. 58

Fig. 59

2. Now lean back, bend your right knee and thigh, straighten your left leg and raise your left toes, keeping your heel on the ground. Turn your body back and 45 degrees to the right. Grasp the stick and bring it back to your abdomen in an arc, roll it up to your chest and turn your wrist (Figs. 60 and 61). Then settle your left foot, and move your weight forward again into a left bow stance. Now clamp the stick and push it upward, to the front and downward until it ends at waist height, as if rowing with an oar. Eyes follow the direction of the stick (Figs. 58 and 59).

Repeat.

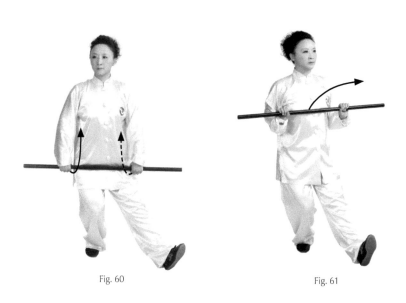

Fig. 60 Fig. 61

3. Move your weight back, bend your right knee and extend your left leg again. Arch your left toes up and keep your heel on the ground. Hold the stick and draw it to your abdomen with an arc, then roll it up to your chest (Figs. 60 and 61). Bring your feet together, shift your weight back and stand erect. At the same time, push the stick outward and pull it back to your abdomen (Figs. 62 and 63).

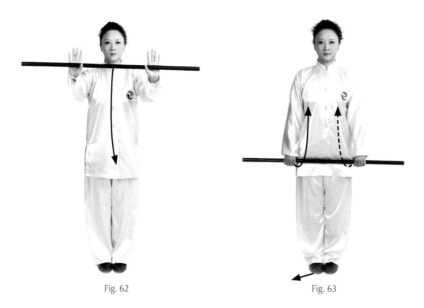

Fig. 62   Fig. 63

The movements on the right side mirror those on the left in the opposite direction (Figs. 64 to 70).

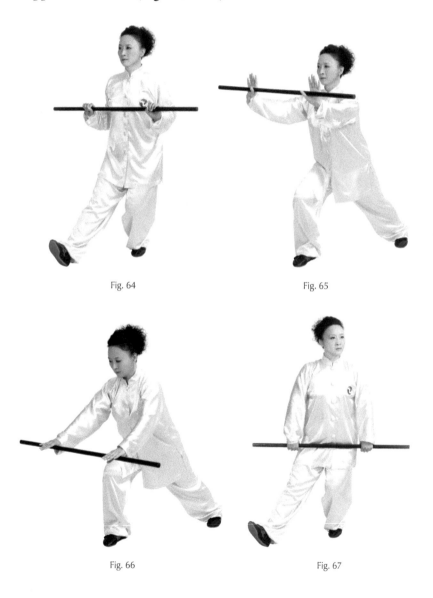

Fig. 64

Fig. 65

Fig. 66

Fig. 67

39

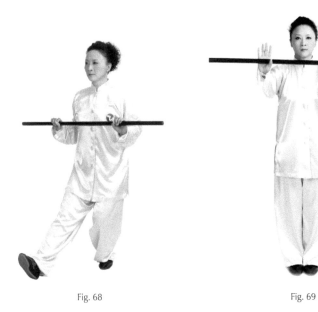

Fig. 68   Fig. 69

Tips

1. When you step forward to form a bow stance, choose a length of stride appropriate to your physical condition. You should make the move gradually and do not stick the hips up.

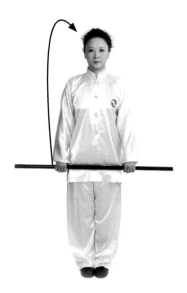

Fig. 70

2. When you move the stick in front of your body, your arms and legs should synchronize naturally and smoothly. You should keep the stick moving between your shoulders and waist, and your elbows and shoulders should move as you push the stick forward. Keep your elbows bent naturally, crane your neck to lift the *Baihui* acupoint upward and breathe deeply.

Health benefits

1. Regular movements of the wrists can stimulate the acupuncture points on the wrists, clear the Hand-*Shaoyin* heart meridian, Hand-*Jueyin* pericardium meridian, and the Hand-*Taiyin* lung meridian, nurturing the heart and calming the nerves (see Appendix: Acupuncture Points).

2. Regular movements of the wrists help ease and reduce the excessive stress of your muscles and tendons from work and daily life.

Step 2 Boat Rows Slowly (*Qing Zhou Huan Xing*)
Movements

1. Continue from "Boatman Rows with an Oar." Bend your knees and step your left foot directly forward. Arch your toes and instep back and stick your heel to the ground. Turn your waist right, hold the stick with both hands and draw an arc from the right side, above your head (Fig. 71-1). Then spread your right hand, turn 180 degrees left with the right palm up and the stick resting on it (Fig. 71-2). Move your weight forward, straighten your knees, set your left foot flat on the ground and touch the

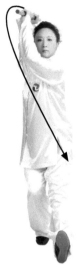
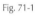
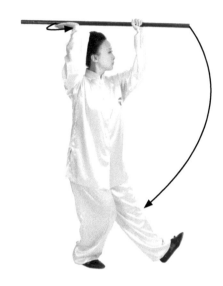

Fig. 71-1   Fig. 71-2

ground with your right toes. Turn your waist 45 degrees to the left. Draw a curve with the stick to the front, side and back of your body until the right hand rests on your left side at the waist, like rowing a boat. Look straight ahead (Fig. 72).

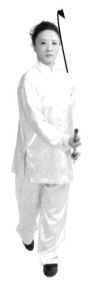

Fig. 72

2. Shift your weight backward, bend your right knee and thigh, and then extend your left leg naturally. At the same time, turn your waist further to the left, hold the stick in both hands and draw an arc from the left side, ending above your head (Fig. 73-1). Then spread your right palm, turn 180 degrees with palm up and rest the stick on it (Fig. 73-2). Step the left foot back along the right ankle, bend your left knee and thigh, and extend your right leg naturally. Arch your right toes back and stick the heel to the ground. Turn your waist 45 degrees to the right, draw an arc with the stick from the side and back of your body until the right hand rests on your right side at the waist as if rowing a boat. Look straight ahead (Fig. 74).

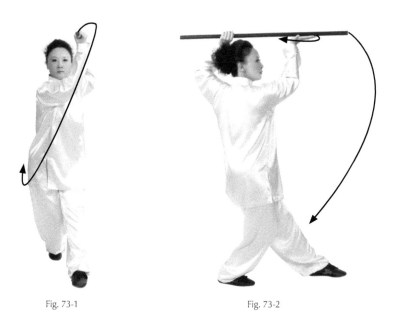

Fig. 73-1   Fig. 73-2

3. Put your feet together and bend your knees. At the same time, turn your waist to the right, hold the stick in both hands and draw an arc from the right side, above your head (Fig. 75). Then straighten your knees, stand upright and turn your waist 45 degrees to the left. Draw an arc from behind your body forward until the right hand rests on your left side at the waist as if rowing a boat. Look straight ahead (Fig. 76).

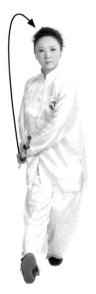

Fig. 74

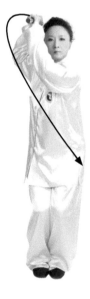

Fig. 75

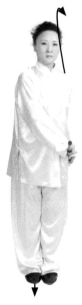

Fig. 76

Movements to the right side mirror those to the left in the opposite direction (Figs. 77 to 82).

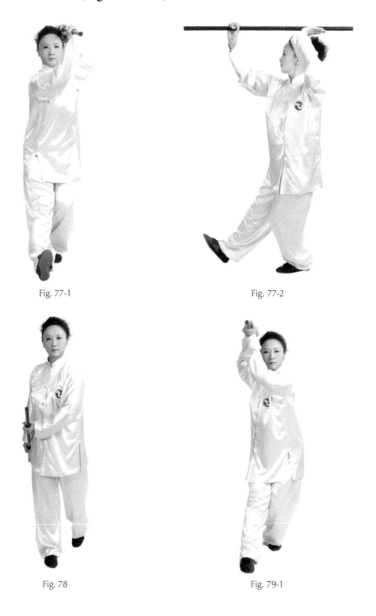

Fig. 77-1   Fig. 77-2

Fig. 78   Fig. 79-1

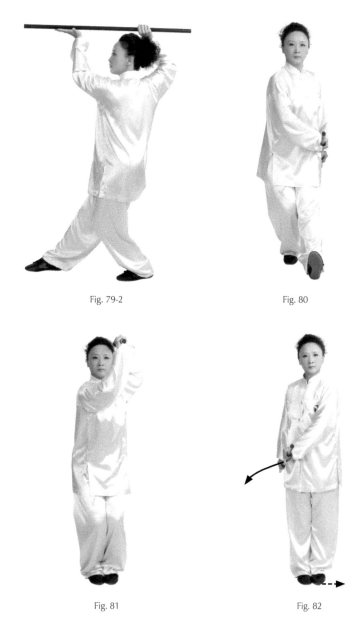

Fig. 79-2   Fig. 80

Fig. 81   Fig. 82

This movement should be done once on each side.

Tips

1. When you "draw a circle" around your body, you should turn your waist naturally and flow with the stick motion; your eyes should follow the moving stick; inhale when gathering momentum and exhale when completing the motion.

2. When you hold the stick, imagine transferring strength downward along the stick, and drop the *qi* to the *Dantian*.

3. Beginners may expand the space between their feet when stepping up or back. When your skills advance and your balance improves, the inside of the feet should be on a line.

4. A practitioner with shoulder problems should have special training for these movements, and control their speed and range.

Health benefits

1. The motion of rowing an oar helps your wrists and shoulders rotate to stimulate the Hand-*Sanyin* and Hand-*Sanyang* meridians, i.e. the coordination of the lung meridian with the large intestine meridian, the heart meridian with the small intestine meridian, the pericardium meridian with the *Sanjiao* meridian. This set of movements promotes digestion and intestinal health.

2. Ankle movements stimulate the Foot-*Sanyin* meridian and the Foot-*Sanyang* meridian, and also regulate the functions of the liver, gallbladder and urine bladder.

3. Rotation of the shoulders helps prevent and cure shoulder arthritis and lessen shoulder pain.

Step 3 Wind Kisses Lotus Leaves (*Feng Bai He Ye*)

Movements

1. Continue from "Boat Rows Slowly." Step your left foot out to the side, with feet parallel and shoulder-width apart. Bend the knees slowly and deeply. Turn your waist 45 degrees to the left, then clamp the stick between thumb and index finger with your palms facing down. Now draw a horizontal circle to the left in front of your abdomen (Figs. 83 and 83). Straighten your knees and stand naturally, roll your wrists, and draw the stick back against your body. Look forward and to the left (Fig. 85).

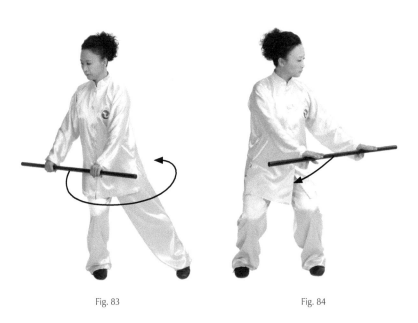

Fig. 83   Fig. 84

2. Without moving your legs, turn your waist to the right, massage across the abdomen from left to right, and raise the stick with your right hand up to the back of your right shoulder, hold the stick with your left hand resting above the right waist (Fig. 86). Then bend your knees deeply; center your waist and draw circles with both hands in opposite directions; end with your arms folded in front of your chest with your right arm up, and looking straight ahead (Fig. 87).

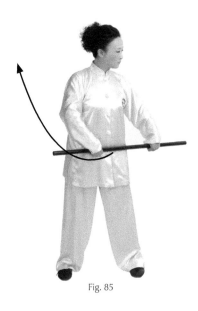

Fig. 85

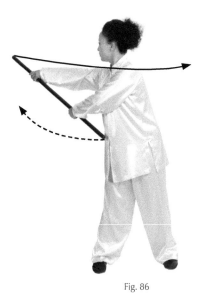

Fig. 86

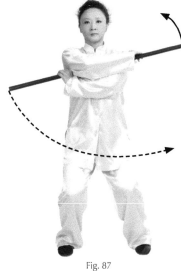

Fig. 87

3. Straighten your knees and stand naturally; hold the stick in your left hand and draw a circle, passing the waist, toward the left until parallel with the left heel, left foot at the height of the waist. Straighten the right arm naturally and place it beside the right ear. The body bends left with the stick extending obliquely and slightly back on the left side (Fig. 88). Relax your fingers and clamp the stick. Look in the direction of the stick (Fig. 89).

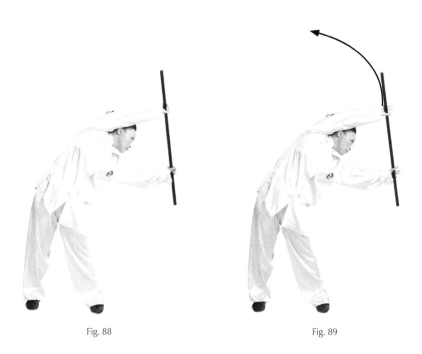

Fig. 88 Fig. 89

4. Without moving your feet, stand upright and lift your head, raise the stick up over your head and straighten your wrists with fingers up. Extend your arms further upward, and look up (Fig. 90). Then bend your knees, lower the stick to your chest, roll it down to your abdomen with palms down. Bring your feet together, and stand upright. Look straight ahead (Figs. 91 and 92).

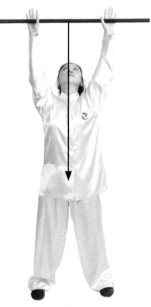

Fig. 90

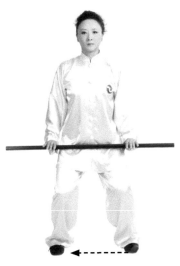

Fig. 91

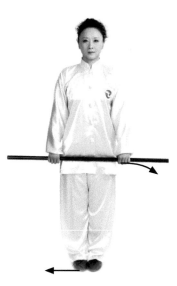

Fig. 92

Movements to the right side mirror the left side in opposite direction (Figs. 93 to 102).

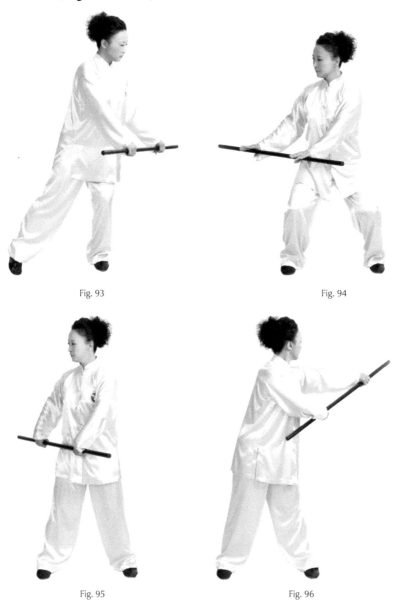

Fig. 93

Fig. 94

Fig. 95

Fig. 96

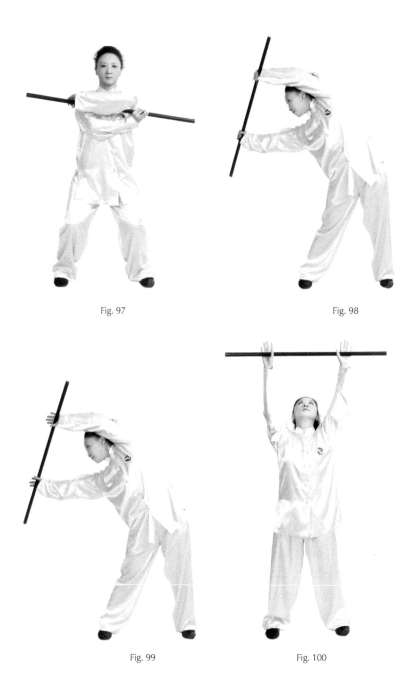

Fig. 97

Fig. 98

Fig. 99

Fig. 100

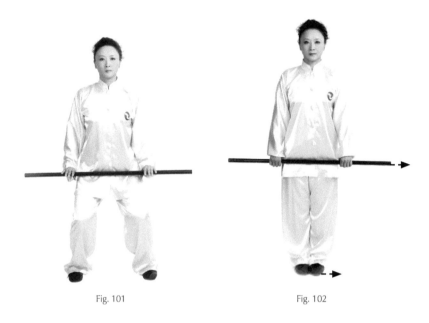

Fig. 101   Fig. 102

This set of movements is done on each side and repeated twice.

Tips

1. In this set, you should coordinate your wrist movements in different ways of holding the stick.

2. When you hold the stick and draw circles in both directions, relax your shoulders and extend your arms as you turn your waist.

3. When you bend the body and draw circles with the stick, the hand at the lower end of the stick guides the movement and must remain no higher than the waist; the arm holding the other end should remain high, near the ear. The priority for each hand should be the smooth movement of the stick.

4. Older people may move less forcefully when bending their bodies; young people should use greater force.

5. Adjust the width of your stance according to the length of the stick, your height and weight, and your physical condition.

Health benefits

1. Bending the body helps stimulate the gallbladder meridian, the *Chong* meridian channel and the *Ren* and *Du* meridian channels, regulates your liver and gallbladder, suppresses liver *yang* hyperactivity, and promotes unblocked circulation of blood and *qi*.

2. According to chiropractic theory, bending the spinal column can also help prevent or adjust spinal asymmetry, effectively preventing deformity.

Step 4 Boatman Tows a Boat (*Chuan Fu Bei Qian*)
Movements

1. Continuing from the previous exercise, step your left foot out to the side, turn your body to the left, and bend your knees into a bow stance; push the stick to the left, draw a circle downward, forward and upward, then pull the upper end to your waist on the left side and point the lower end forward. Look ahead and to the left (Figs. 103 to 105).

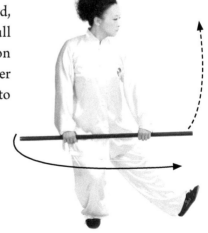

Fig. 103

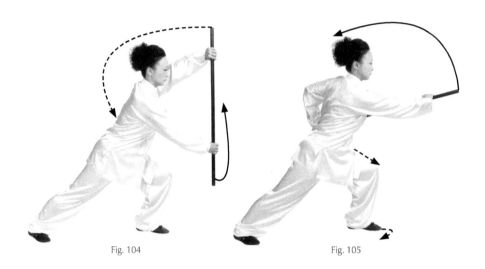

Fig. 104   Fig. 105

2. Shift your weight to the right, turn your right sole outward, plant your left foot inward, with feet parallel, straighten your knees as you stand up. Turn your waist to the right, push the stick downward with your left hand, then forward, passing the outside of left knee, to draw a circle upward; the right hand, holding the stick, draws a circle backward, rightward and downward, and then presses the stick on your shoulders, looking ahead (Fig. 106).

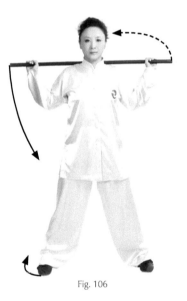

Fig. 106

3. Turn the right foot 90 degrees outward, extend the left foot to left rear, and bend the right knee into a bow stance; at the same time, turn your waist to the right, and massage your shoulder with the stick while rotating it 180 degrees (Figs 107 and 108); lower your weight further, press the *Jianjing* acupoint on your left shoulder with the stick; look back to the right and rear (Fig. 109).

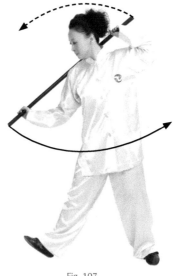

Fig. 107

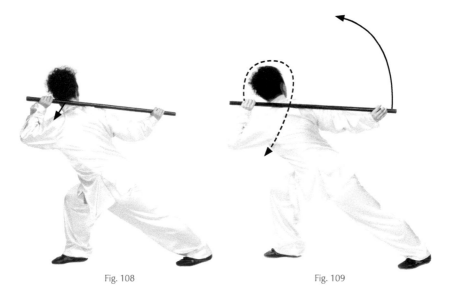

Fig. 108

Fig. 109

4. Push the stick above your head with your left hand, then lower it to your right shoulder and then to your right chest, then draw an arc upward with the stick end with your right hand (Fig. 110); shift your weight to the left, turn your left foot out and bend the left knee, turning the right foot inward and extending the right leg. Turn your body back and wield the stick in an arc across your abdomen to the left (Fig. 111); shift your weight to your right leg, bending the knee. Then bring your feet together and bend your knees, pushing the stick up above your head with your fingers pointed up and hands clamping the stick; then straighten your legs and stand upright, lowering the stick to your chest and then abdomen. Hold the stick in front of your abdomen and look straight ahead (Figs. 112 and 113).

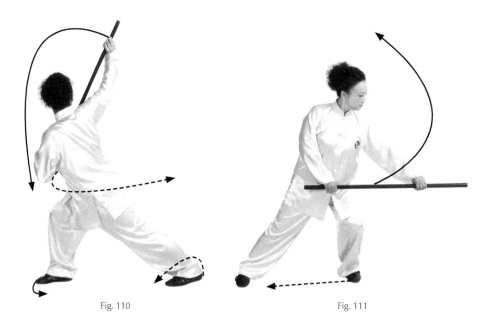

Fig. 110   Fig. 111

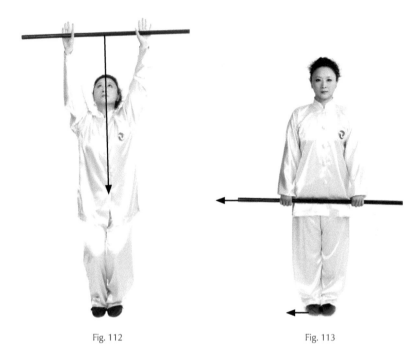

Fig. 112   Fig. 113

Movements to the right side mirror those on the left side in the opposite direction (Figs. 114 to 124).

This set of movements is repeated twice on each side.

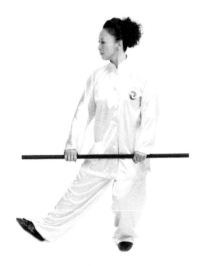

Fig. 114

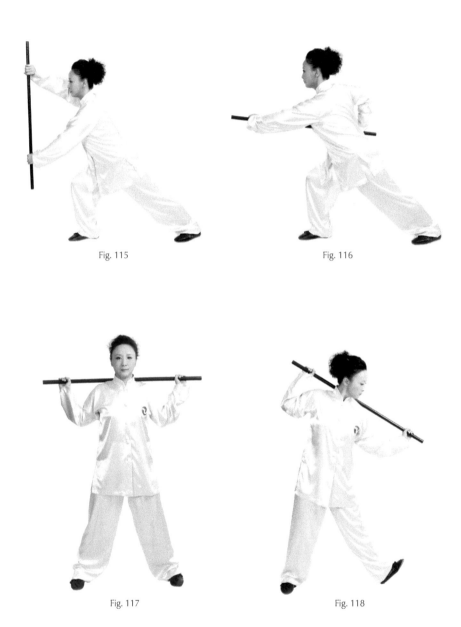

Fig. 115

Fig. 116

Fig. 117

Fig. 118

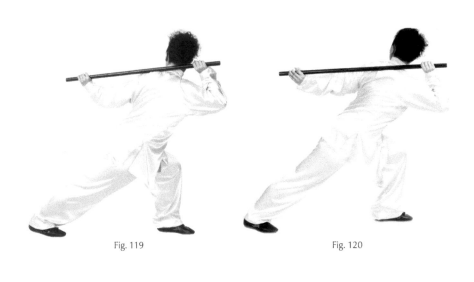

Fig. 119

Fig. 120

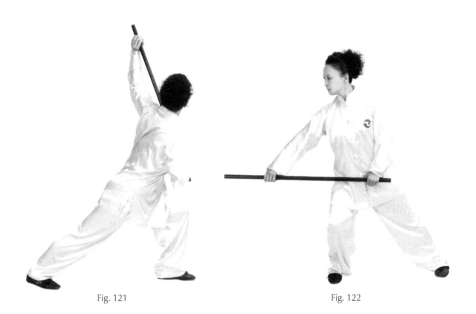

Fig. 121

Fig. 122

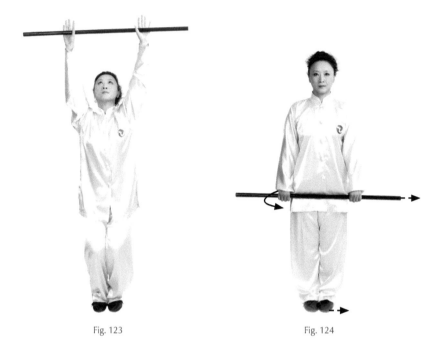

Fig. 123   Fig. 124

Tips

1. Use "rotating the stick to the left" as an example. When you draw curves upward and to the left, your left hand should slide slightly toward the end of the stick, as you straighten your knees and stand up; when you rotate the stick and press it on your shoulder, your right hand should slide to the end of the stick, with your hands in symmetrical positions.

2. When you hold the stick and draw curves behind you, your waist should rotate and extend as well.

3. When you turn your waist leftward and rotate the stick, you should slide the stick on your shoulder as you turn your waist, and then draw circles on the side and behind your back. Your right

hand should cooperate with your left, with your stick rotating approximately 180 degrees.

4. When you turn your waist and shoulders, you should rotate the stick after you stop. Beginners should shift their weight higher, keep their stride short, and turn their bodies slightly. You may keep your stride bigger, turn your waist and extend your legs to the full until your upper body and legs are in line when you become more skilled.

5. When you massage your shoulders with the stick, do so gently. When you turn your waist to the right, you should press the *Jianjing* acupoint on the left shoulder and vice versa. Also, remember to coordinate your movements with your breathing.

Health benefits

1. Turning your head can effectively stimulate the *Dazhui* acupoint, invigorate the *qi* and strengthen *yang*; pressing the *Jianjing* acupoint helps promote the circulation of blood and *qi* and strengthen the body; it also relieves rheumatism, drives off coldness, and reduces pain in your neck, shoulders and back.

2. Turning your waist, straightening your legs and stretching your feet can further stimulate the *Ren* and *Du* meridian channels, the *Dai* meridian channel, and the Foot-*Sanyin* and Foot-*Sanyang* meridians, promote the circulation of blood and *qi*, invigorate your kidneys and strengthen *yang*. These movements also help increase the flexibility of your lumbar vertebrae and hip joints, and stretch the muscle groups of the waist and legs, thereby improving their flexibility and agility.

Step 5 Iron Stick Calms the Sea (*Shen Zhen Ding Hai*)

Movements

1. Continue from "Boatman Tows a Boat." Bend your knees slightly. Shift your weight to the left, with feet parallel and shoulder-width apart. Then stand naturally straight; clamp the stick with the left hand, palm down; the right wrist rotates outward and holds the stick with palm up. Draw a vertical circle above your head (Figs. 125 and 126); then bend your knees deeply and lower the stick along your side to waist height; your eyes follow the direction of the stick (Fig. 127).

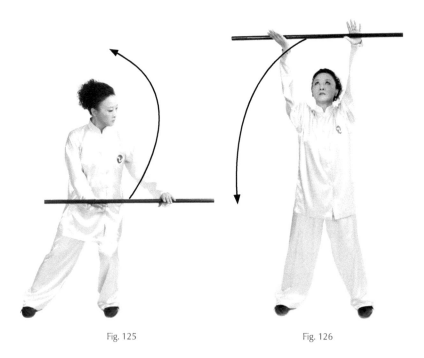

Fig. 125   Fig. 126

2. Straighten your legs and turn your waist slightly to the right; rotate the stick with your left hand, holding it in front of your chest with your right palm cradling the extended end (Fig. 128); then turn your left foot 90 degrees outward, stretch your right foot to right back, bending your knees into a bow stance; at the same time, turn your body left, and draw a curve in front of your body; look straight ahead (Fig. 129).

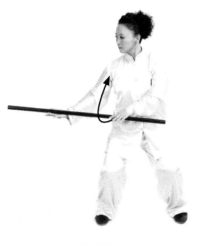

Fig. 127

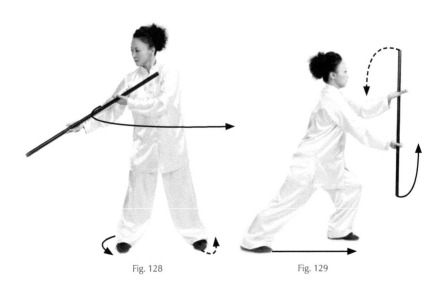

Fig. 128

Fig. 129

3. Bring your right foot forward, so your feet are parallel and shoulder-width apart. Bend your knees deeply; push the end of the stick nearest your chest downward with your left hand until it reaches waist height, while your right hand slides slightly to the right end of the stick and then pulls it upward until the stick is held vertically in front of your body with your right hand at eye level (Figs. 130 and 131); then slide the right hand down until it meets the left hand; look straight ahead (Fig. 132).

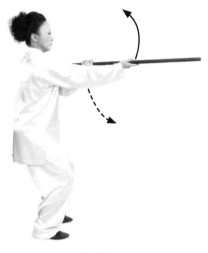

Fig. 130

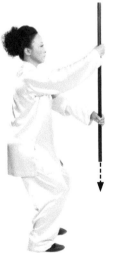

Fig. 131

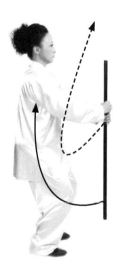

Fig. 132

4. Straighten your knees and stand upright; the hands fall down to the front of the abdomen and separate. Straighten the arms by the sides of the body, with the right hand holding the stick after you turn it 180 degrees to move in an arc to the rear and upward to place it behind your right arm; extend your left arm at 45 degrees to the left front at face height, palms up (Fig. 133); then relax your thighs, slightly bend your knees; bend your left elbow, with palm facing down, and place the palm in front of the abdomen, and look straight ahead (Figs. 134 and 135).

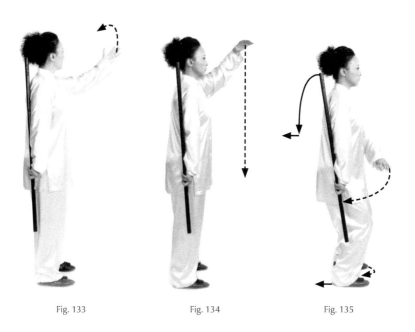

Fig. 133   Fig. 134   Fig. 135

Movements to the right side
mirror those on the left side in
the opposite direction (Figs.
136 to 146).

This set of movements is
done on each side once and
repeated twice.

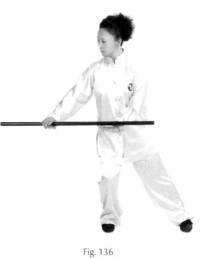

Fig. 136

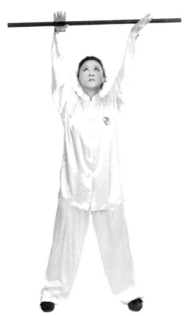

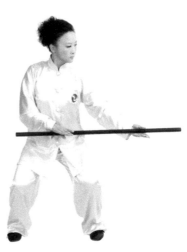

Fig. 137

Fig. 138

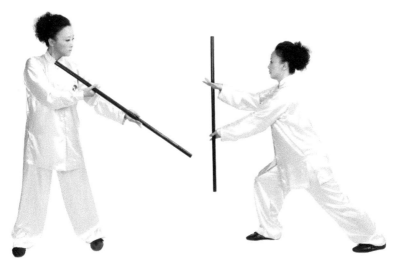

Fig. 139   Fig. 140

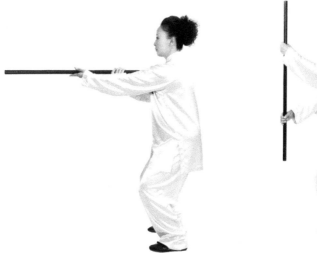

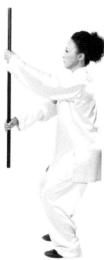

Fig. 141   Fig. 142

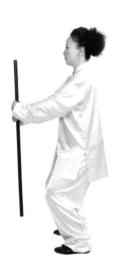

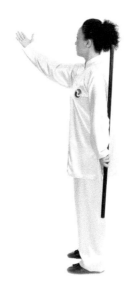

Fig. 143

Fig. 144

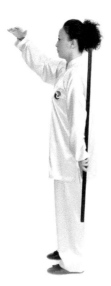

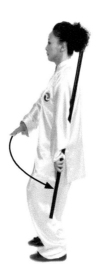

Fig. 145

Fig. 146

Tips

1. When you cannot manage the stick well, try practicing some basic movements such as rotating, rolling and sliding the stick.

2. Coordinate your breathing with the movements. As your skills advance, your breath will become deep and light, primarily abdominal breathing.

3. When you lift your arm and extend your hand, relax your shoulders, bend your elbow, imagine you are breathing the essence of nature deep into your *Dantian*, and stand quietly for a moment.

Health benefits

1. Wrist rotation makes up for the lack of such movements in daily life, and helps effectively to prevent wrist injury.

2. Guiding the movement of *qi* with the stick, and imagining the absorption of nature's essence into your *Dantian* from the *Baihui* acupoint, to nurture the soul, help maintain your vitality and improve the effect of the exercise.

Step 6 Golden Dragon Wags Its Tail (*Jin Long Jiao Wei*)

Movements

1. Continue from the previous sequence. Turn your right foot inward, and step your left foot out to your left rear at 45 degrees; hold the stick with your right hand and point it 45 degrees to the right. Move your left hand a third of the way along the stick (Figs. 147 and 148). Shift your weight to the left and pivot your left foot outward and right foot inward, bending the legs into a bow stance to the left; at the same time, turn your body to the left. Draw a vertical circle in front of your body and stop when the stick is at shoulder height, with both hands holding the stick and resting it under the right armpit; gaze at the far end of the stick (Fig. 149).

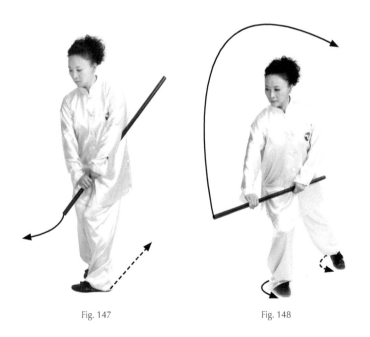

Fig. 147   Fig. 148

2. Shift your weight back onto the right leg, bend your right knee and straighten the left leg; at the same time, slide your left hand forward along the stick and your right hand backward, until the left hand reaches the end of the stick, a bit higher than the left shoulder, and the right hand is near your waist (Fig. 150); then move your left foot across and behind the right, bending both knees; turn right at the waist and look to the front right (Fig. 151).

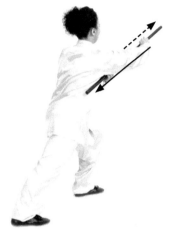

Fig. 149

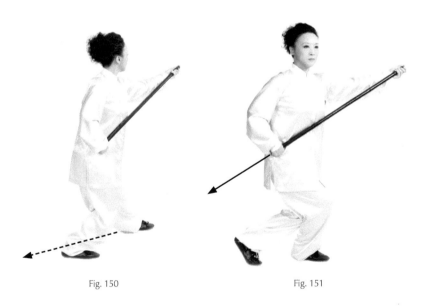

Fig. 150

Fig. 151

3. Lower your weight, bend your knees and squat; turn your waist to the right, extend the stick to the right and front with the left hand at one end till the other end touches the ground; then slide the right hand along the stick a third of its length, and clamp it, looking at the far end of the stick (Fig. 152, older people may squat higher here); then stir with and push the stick along the floor with your palms facing down; look at the stick (Fig. 153).

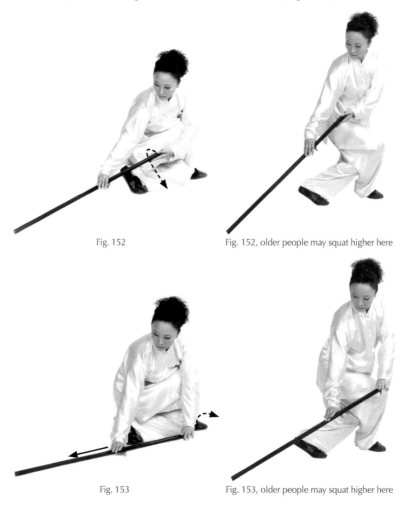

Fig. 152   Fig. 152, older people may squat higher here

Fig. 153   Fig. 153, older people may squat higher here

4. Stand up erect, move your left foot one step to the left, and at the same time slide your left hand to the end of the stick, and your right hand a third of the way along it (Fig. 154). Shift your weight to the left, bring your feet parallel and shoulder-width apart, and stand naturally erect; move your left hand a third of the way along the stick, and grasp it in front of your abdomen; look straight ahead (Fig. 155).

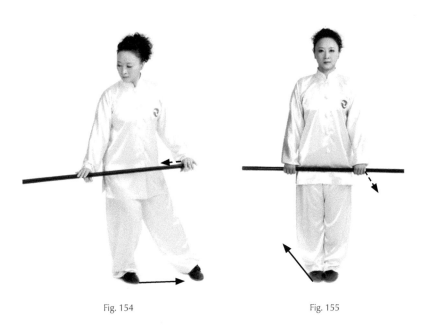

Fig. 154   Fig. 155

Movements to the right side mirror those on the left in the opposite direction (Figs. 156 to 163). Older people can take a higher squat pose (Figs. 160 and 161).

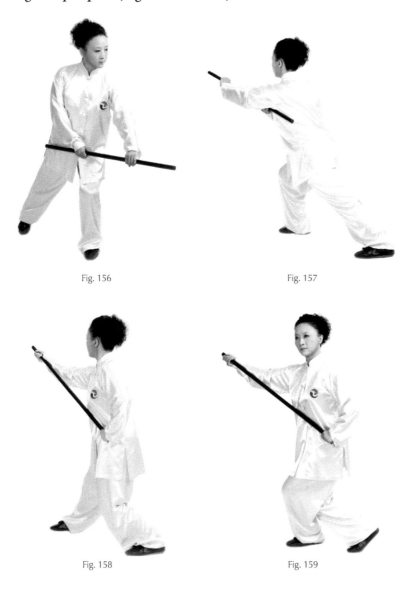

Fig. 156   Fig. 157

Fig. 158   Fig. 159

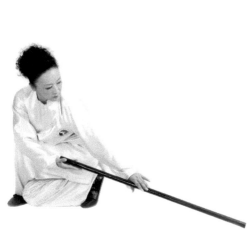

Fig. 160

Fig. 160, older people may squat higher here

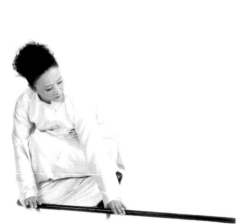

Fig. 161

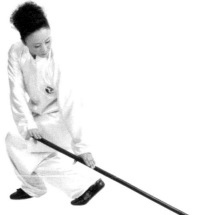

Fig. 161, older people may squat higher here

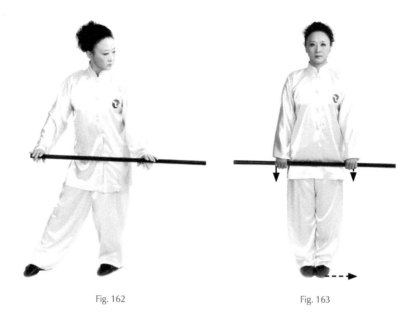

Fig. 162   Fig. 163

This set of movements is done on each side once and repeated twice.

Tips

1. The balance of *yin* and *yang* should be manifested in every movement of this set of exercises. When you push the stick forward, you extend your legs backward; as you draw a vertical circle from the bottom up, you move your weight downward.

2. When you twist the stick, rotate your wrists outward and inhale at the same time; as you press the stick, rotate your wrists inward and exhale; when you rise and spread your feet apart, you inhale; when you bring your feet together and sink with bending knees, you exhale.

3. Older people with high blood pressure or heart disease may choose a higher squat with one knee pressed against *Chengshan* acupoint of the other leg. Younger people should choose the lower squat. As the physical condition of the older practitioner improves, the low squat becomes an option.

4. When you draw a vertical circle, relax your shoulders and stretch your arms; when you slide your hands to the ends of the stick, you should hold the stick tight, lowering your shoulders and elbows.

Health benefits

1. When bending the knees with one knee pressed against the *Chengshan* acupoint of the other leg, you stimulate the Foot-*Taiyang* bladder meridian effectively. This regulates the flow of urine, as the bladder meridian channel is connected with the kidney channel.

2. Rotating your body from the waist helps stimulate the *Dai* meridian channel, which is responsible for thorough circulation in the meridians, and is good for the smooth flow of *qi* throughout the body.

3. Squatting demands flexibility and the ability to balance and control the strength in your legs. Squatting helps strengthen older people's leg muscles, improve their balancing ability and reduce muscle spasm and cramping.

Step 7 Search for Treasure in the Sea (*Tan Hai Xun Bao*)

Movements

1. Continue from the last step. Step out with your left foot, parallel to and shoulder-width apart from the right, and stand naturally straight; push the stick to shoulder height, then pull it back to your chest, and roll it down over the body to your feet. Keep your arms straight and your eyes on the stick (Figs. 164 to 166).

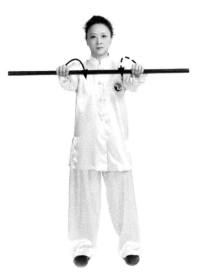

Fig. 164

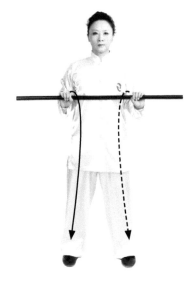

Fig. 165

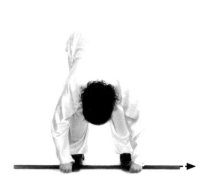

Fig. 166

2. Bend your knees slightly and then extend, shifting your weight to your left leg; then turn your head and body to the left, pushing the stick leftward and then upward until your right hand comes to left shoulder height; watch the upper end of the stick (Figs. 167 and 168); then shift your weight to the right, turn your body and head back, and arch your back slightly, lowering the stick to the ground in front of your feet, with your eyes focused on the stick (Fig. 169).

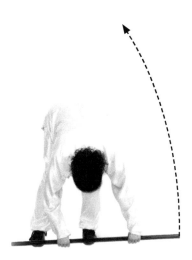

Fig. 167

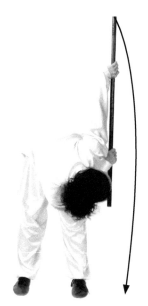

Fig. 168

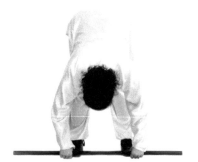

Fig. 169

3. Straighten your legs; keep the deep bend in the back, drop your arms naturally with the stick nearly on the floor, then raise your head, taking and exhaling a breath; look straight ahead (Figs. 170-1 and 170-2).

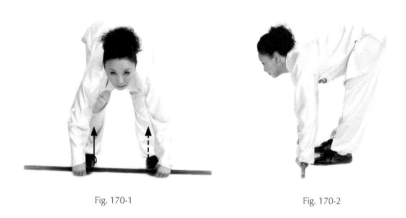

Fig. 170-1   Fig. 170-2

4. Stand erect, rolling the stick up over your legs to your chest (Fig. 171); bring your feet together and stand naturally erect; roll the stick down to your abdomen with full arm extension; look straight ahead (Fig. 172).

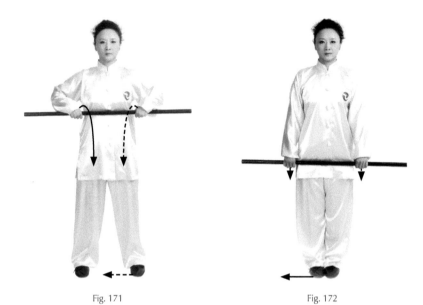

Fig. 171

Fig. 172

Movements to the right side mirror those on the left side in the opposite direction (Figs. 173 to 181).

This set of movements is done once on each side and repeated twice.

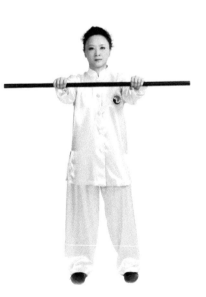

Fig. 173

Chapter IV
Movements

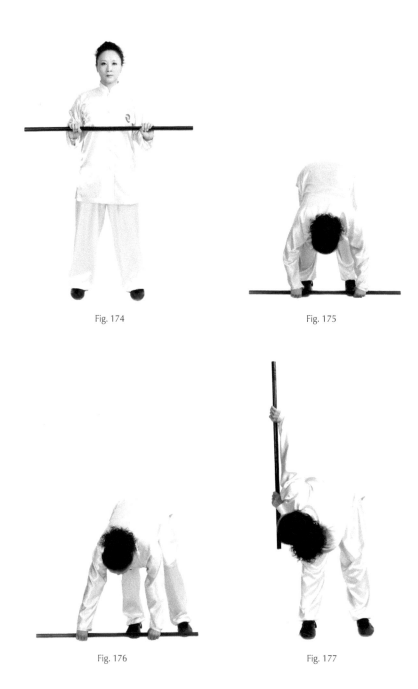

Fig. 174

Fig. 175

Fig. 176

Fig. 177

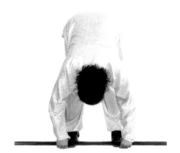

Fig. 178

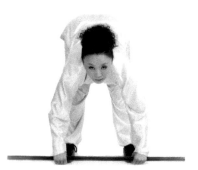

Fig. 179

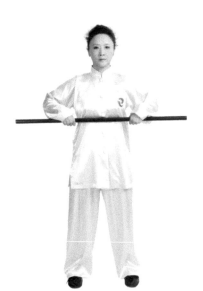

Fig. 180

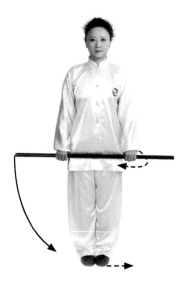

Fig. 181

Tips

1. When you raise the stick in front of your body, lower your shoulders and raise your elbows; when you draw the stick back to your chest, flex your hands, wrists and elbows in succession.

2. When you bend your back and turn your body leftward, your left hand guides the stick and the right hand follows; when you turn your body to the right, bend your back and lower the stick, drop the right hand first and then the left.

3. Your breath should be light but deep, in harmony with your movements, relying primarily on abdominal breathing.

4. Beginners and older people should not bend too low; avoid constricted breathing and pressure in your chest. Keep your knees straight and your breathing smooth.

Health benefits

1. Turning your body and head, and raising your head and bending your back effectively stimulate the *Dai* meridian channel, and the *Ren* and *Du* meridian channels. This helps promote the circulation of blood and *qi*, invigorate the kidneys and strengthen the abdomen to improve your health.

2. Bending your knees and back helps stretch the muscle groups of your legs, improving flexibility and lessening the fatigue and tension of the muscles in your back.

Step 8 *Qi* Returns to *Dantian* (*Qi Gui Dan Tian*)

Movements

1. Continue from the last sequence. Open you left palm and hold the stick with palms down; turn your wrists outward, clamp the rod vertically, and let your arms hang naturally at your sides; step out your left foot, with feet parallel and shoulder-width apart. Stand naturally straight, and look straight ahead (Fig. 182).

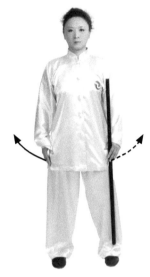

Fig. 182

2. Bend your knees; hold your arms in front of your abdomen, with palms facing inside and fingers pointing each other, 10 cm apart; look straight ahead and hold this pose (Figs. 183 and 184).

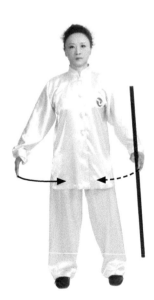

Fig. 183

87

3. Stand upright again; bring your hands down to the front of the *Dantian*, then let your arms hang naturally at your sides; look straight ahead (Fig. 185).

Repeat 2 and 3 twice.

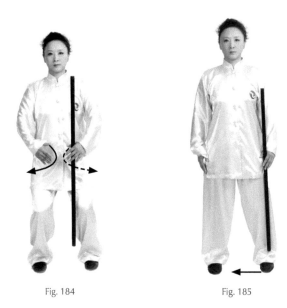

Fig. 184   Fig. 185

Tips

When you bring your hands in front of the *Dantian*, your hands should be 10 cm apart, and then separate your arms to let them hang.

Health benefits

Guiding the flow of *qi* with imagination helps enhance vitality.

Ending Stance

Movements

Continuing from the last step, pause, bring your feet together, and stand naturally straight; look straight ahead, and hold the stick at your side (Fig. 186).

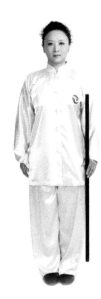

Fig. 186

Tips

1. When you stand up, relax your waist, tighten your hips, raise your elbows, lower your shoulders, stand straight and relax; imagine you are at one with nature.

2. Coordinate your movements with light but deep abdominal breathing. The depth of breath should be natural and varies individually.

Health benefits

Shifting from dynamic flow to the static conclusion consolidates your vitality, and regulates body and mind to the most relaxed and balanced state, to improve your health.

Acupuncture Points

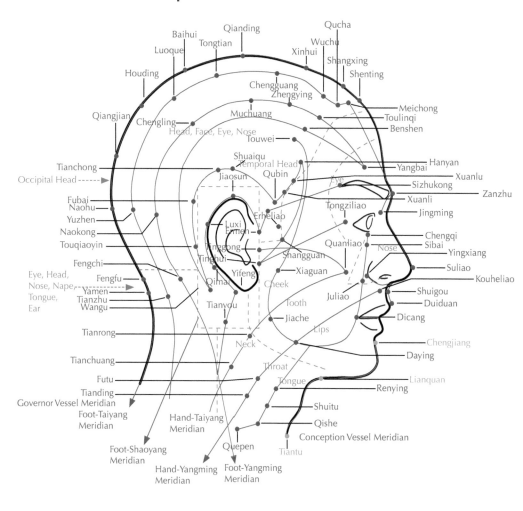

Acupoints on the head and face

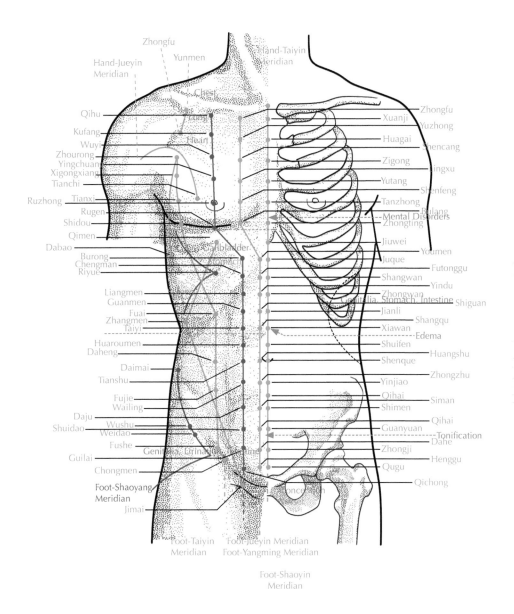

Acupoints on the chest and abdomen

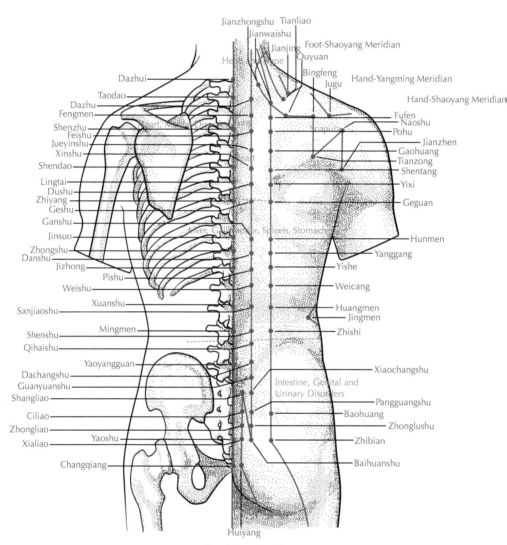

Acupoints on the back and lumbar region

Tianfu
Xiabai
Chize
Quze
Shaohai
Chest, Lung, Throat
Kongzhui
Ximen
Jianshi
Neiguan
Lieque
Jingqu
Taiyuan
Yuji
Shaoshang
Hand-Taiyin Meridian
Hand-Jueyin Meridian
Zhongchong

Tianquan
Disorders at the Medial Region of the Arm
Qingling
Chest, Heart, Mental Disorders
Chest, Heart, Stomach
Chest, Heart, Throat

Lingdao
Tongli
Yinxi
Shenmen
Daling
Shaofu
Laogong

Shaochong
Hand-Shaoyin Meridian

Jianzhen
Jianliao
Jianyu
Naohui
Binao
Xiaoluo
Shouwuli
Qinglengyuan
Tianjing
Xiaohai
Zhouliao
Quchi
Shousanli
Shanglian
Xialian
Head, Face, Nose, Mouth, Tooth, Throat
Sidu
Wenliu
Zhizheng
Sanyangluo
Huizong
Pianli
Zhigou
Wanguan
Yanglao
Yangxi
Yanggu
Yangchi
Wangu
Hegu
Zhongdu
Houxi
Sanjian
Qiangu
Erjian
Yemen
Hand-Yangming Meridian

Shaoze
Shangyang
Guanchong
Hand-Taiyang Meridian

Disorders at the Lateral Region of the Arm
Lateral Head, Chest, Back

Hand-Shaoyang Meridian

Acupoints in the upper limbs

93

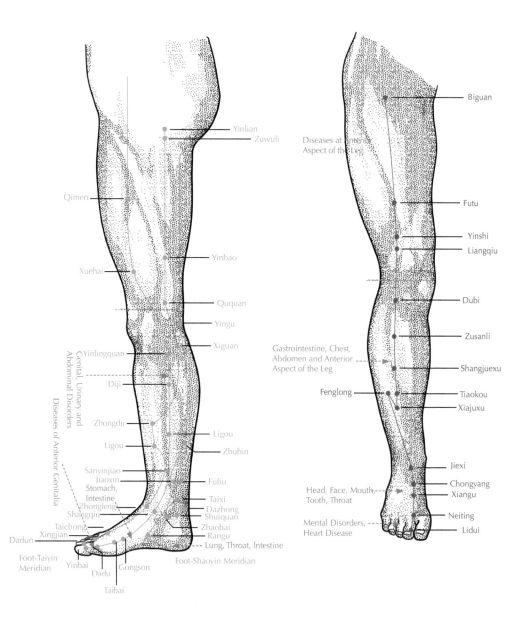

Yinlian
Zuwuli
Qimen
Yinbao
Xuehai
Ququan
Yingu
Xiguan
Yinlingquan
Genital, Urinary and
Abdominal Disorders
Diji
Diseases of Anterior Genitalia
Zhongdu
Ligou
Ligou
Zhubin
Sanyinjiao
Jiaoxin
Fuliu
Stomach,
Intestine
Taixi
Zhongfeng
Dazhong
Shangqiu
Shuiquan
Taichong
Zhaohai
Xingjian
Rangu
Dadun
Foot-Taiyin
Meridian
Yinbai
Dadu
Gongson
Taibai
Lung, Throat, Intestine
Foot-Shaoyin Meridian

Biguan
Diseases at Anterior
Aspect of the Leg
Futu
Yinshi
Liangqiu
Dubi
Zusanli
Gastrointestine, Chest,
Abdomen and Anterior
Aspect of the Leg
Shangjuexu
Fenglong
Tiaokou
Xiajuxu
Jiexi
Head, Face, Mouth,
Tooth, Throat
Chongyang
Xiangu
Mental Disorders,
Heart Disease
Neiting
Lidui

Acupoints in the lower limbs

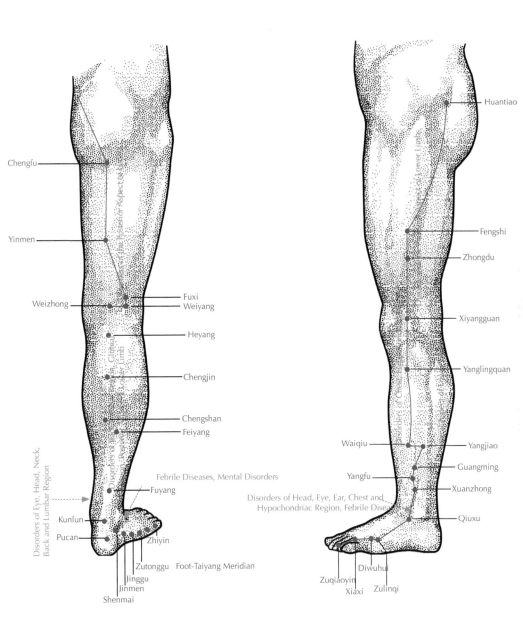

Acupoints in the lower limbs

Taiji Yangsheng Zhang